Rheumatoid Arthritis Diet Cookbook for Women

Essential Nutrition for Managing Symptoms and Boosting Energy

Ennis James

Copyright © 2024 by **Ennis James**
All rights reserved

No part of this publication may be reproduced, stored in a retrieval system, or transmitted, in any form or by any means, electronic, mechanical, photocopying, recording, or otherwise, without the prior written permission of the author.

The information in this ebook is true and complete to the best of our knowledge. All recommendation are made without guarantee on the part of author or publisher. The author and publisher disclaim any liability in connection with the use of this information.

Table of Contents

Introduction

In a quaint suburban neighborhood, lived a woman named Emma. At 45, Emma led a vibrant life filled with family, friends, and a successful career. However, a nagging pain in her joints began to cast a shadow over her days. What started as occasional stiffness soon became debilitating, and she was diagnosed with rheumatoid arthritis.

The diagnosis hit hard. Emma had always been active, running marathons and participating in yoga classes. The thought of being hindered by pain was terrifying. Her doctor prescribed medications, but the side effects left her feeling drained and disheartened. Desperate for a solution, she began researching alternative ways to manage her condition.

One evening, as Emma scrolled through an online forum, she stumbled upon a glowing recommendation for a book titled "Rheumatoid Arthritis Diet Cookbook for Women." The testimonials were compelling; women shared stories of how the book had transformed their lives, reducing their pain and increasing their energy levels.

Intrigued, Emma decided to give it a try. The book promised more than just recipes; it offered a comprehensive guide to understanding how diet could impact rheumatoid arthritis. She ordered it and waited eagerly for it to arrive.

When the book finally came, Emma was immediately impressed by its thoroughness. The introduction explained the science behind rheumatoid arthritis and how certain foods could either exacerbate or alleviate inflammation. The authors had collaborated with nutritionists and medical experts, ensuring the information was accurate and practical.

The first chapter laid out the principles of an arthritis-friendly diet. Emma learned about anti-inflammatory foods and the key nutrients essential for joint health. She was excited to find that many of her favorite foods, like berries, leafy greens, and salmon, were on the list. The book also highlighted foods to avoid, such as refined sugars and processed meats, which could trigger inflammation.

As Emma delved into the breakfast section, she found simple, delicious recipes designed to start her day right. From overnight chia seed pudding with berries to spinach and mushroom omelets, the meals were easy to prepare and packed with nutrients. She decided to try the turmeric golden milk smoothie first, blending the ingredients with care. The result was a creamy, vibrant drink that left her feeling nourished and energized.

For lunch, Emma explored recipes like quinoa and roasted vegetable salad and grilled salmon with steamed greens. The flavors were rich and satisfying, proving that healthy food could also be delicious. Dinner recipes such as baked chicken with sweet potato mash and Mediterranean stuffed bell peppers became new family favorites, enjoyed by her husband and children alike.

Within weeks of following the cookbook's guidelines, Emma noticed significant improvements. Her joint pain decreased, her energy levels soared, and she felt more in control of her health. The book's meal planning tips made it easy to stay organized, and the advice on dining out and traveling helped her maintain her diet even on the go.

Emma's transformation didn't go unnoticed. Friends and family marveled at her renewed vitality and asked about her secret. She eagerly shared her journey and recommended the "Rheumatoid Arthritis Diet Cookbook for Women."

"It's more than just a cookbook," she would say. "It's a lifeline. It empowers you with knowledge and provides delicious, easy-to-make recipes that truly make a difference."

The book had not only improved Emma's physical health but also boosted her emotional well-being. She felt hopeful and inspired, ready to embrace life with newfound confidence. For anyone battling rheumatoid arthritis, this cookbook was a beacon of hope, showing that with the right tools, they could reclaim their lives and thrive.

Rheumatoid arthritis is an autoimmune disease where the body's immune system mistakenly attacks the joints, leading to inflammation, pain, and swelling. Unlike osteoarthritis, which is caused by wear and tear, rheumatoid arthritis results from an immune response that targets the synovium—the lining of the membranes surrounding the joints. This inflammation can eventually cause bone erosion and joint deformity, significantly affecting a person's mobility and quality of life. The condition is chronic, meaning it persists for a long time, often with periods of remission and flare-ups.

Women are more likely to develop rheumatoid arthritis than men, and the symptoms often appear between the ages of 30 and 60. The exact cause is unknown, but a combination of genetic and environmental factors is believed to trigger the onset. Common symptoms include tender, warm, swollen joints, joint stiffness that is usually worse in the mornings and after inactivity, fatigue, fever, and loss of appetite. These symptoms can vary in severity and may affect different parts of the body at different times.

Managing rheumatoid arthritis typically involves a combination of medications, lifestyle changes, and dietary adjustments. While medications like NSAIDs, corticosteroids, and DMARDs can help control inflammation and pain, they often come with side effects. This has led many individuals to seek complementary approaches to managing their condition, such as dietary changes. Research suggests that certain foods can either exacerbate or help reduce the symptoms of rheumatoid arthritis.

The rheumatoid arthritis diet focuses on anti-inflammatory foods that can help manage symptoms and improve overall health. This includes incorporating omega-3 fatty acids found in fish, flaxseeds, and walnuts, which have been shown to reduce inflammation. Fruits and vegetables rich in antioxidants, such as berries, spinach, and kale, help combat oxidative stress, a contributor to chronic inflammation. Whole grains, lean proteins, and healthy fats are also essential components of this diet, providing necessary nutrients without triggering inflammatory responses.

Conversely, some foods can worsen inflammation and should be limited or avoided. These include processed foods high in sugar and unhealthy fats, red and processed meats, and refined carbohydrates. Such foods can increase inflammatory markers in the body, potentially leading to flare-ups and increased joint pain. The rheumatoid arthritis diet cookbook for women provides detailed guidance on which foods to embrace and which to avoid, helping to make meal planning simpler and more effective.

Implementing a rheumatoid arthritis-friendly diet requires a commitment to healthy eating habits and meal preparation.

The cookbook offers practical advice on creating balanced, nutritious meals that align with the dietary needs of someone managing rheumatoid arthritis. It includes recipes that are easy to follow, delicious, and specifically designed to reduce inflammation and support joint health. By adhering to these dietary principles, women with rheumatoid arthritis can experience a reduction in symptoms, improved energy levels, and a better quality of life.

The rheumatoid arthritis diet cookbook for women is more than just a collection of recipes; it is a comprehensive guide to understanding how food impacts the condition and how to use nutrition as a powerful tool in managing it. It empowers women to take control of their health through informed dietary choices, offering a pathway to relief and wellness. By integrating these dietary strategies into their daily lives, women can find a sustainable way to live well with rheumatoid arthritis, minimizing its impact on their daily activities and overall well-being.

This cookbook is designed to be a comprehensive guide for women managing rheumatoid arthritis through diet. Each section is thoughtfully crafted to provide not just recipes, but also an understanding of how specific foods can impact your health. Begin by familiarizing yourself with the principles outlined in the early chapters. These sections explain the science behind inflammation and the role of nutrition in managing symptoms. Understanding these fundamentals will help you make informed decisions about your meals.

As you explore the recipes, you'll notice they are divided into categories such as breakfast, lunch, dinner, snacks, and desserts. This organization makes it easy to plan your meals throughout the day. Each recipe includes detailed instructions, ingredient lists, and nutritional information tailored to meet the needs of those with rheumatoid arthritis. Pay attention to the ingredient lists, as they highlight anti-inflammatory foods and avoid common dietary triggers.

When preparing your meals, take note of the cooking tips provided. These tips are especially useful if you are new to cooking or adapting to a different way of eating. The cookbook includes suggestions on how to substitute ingredients, prepare meals in advance, and store leftovers. These practical tips can save time and ensure you always have healthy options available, even on busy days.

The meal planning section is particularly valuable for maintaining consistency in your diet. It offers sample meal plans and shopping lists, which can simplify your grocery trips and help you stay organized. By following these plans, you can ensure that your diet remains balanced and supportive of your health goals. The sample plans are flexible and can be adjusted based on your preferences and lifestyle.

In addition to recipes, the cookbook provides guidance on dining out and traveling. Eating out can be challenging when managing rheumatoid arthritis, but the tips offered will help you make better choices. Look for dishes that align with the principles of an anti-inflammatory diet and don't hesitate to ask for modifications to suit your needs. When traveling, the book suggests packing snacks and planning ahead to maintain your dietary regimen.

Incorporating these recipes into your daily life can lead to significant improvements in your symptoms. Many readers have reported reduced joint pain and increased energy levels after consistently following the guidelines. The key is to approach this lifestyle change with patience and dedication. Over time, you will likely find that these recipes become second nature, making it easier to stick to your diet and enjoy the benefits.

Finally, this cookbook is not just about food; it's about a holistic approach to managing rheumatoid arthritis. Alongside dietary changes, consider incorporating other lifestyle adjustments recommended in the book, such as regular exercise and stress management techniques. By integrating these practices into your routine, you can enhance your overall well-being and improve your quality of life.

Chapter 1: Breakfast Recipes

Overnight Chia Seed Pudding with Berries

Ingredient:

- 1/4 cup chia seeds
- 1 cup unsweetened almond milk (or any preferred milk)
- 1 tablespoon maple syrup or honey
- 1/2 teaspoon vanilla extract
- 1/2 cup mixed berries (blueberries, strawberries, raspberries)

Instructions:

1. In a medium-sized bowl or jar, combine the chia seeds, almond milk, maple syrup or honey, and vanilla extract. Stir well to ensure the chia seeds are evenly distributed.
2. Cover the bowl or jar and refrigerate overnight, or for at least 4 hours.
3. In the morning, give the pudding a good stir. If the consistency is too thick, you can add a little more almond milk to reach your desired consistency.

4. Top with mixed berries and enjoy.

Nutritional Information:

- Calories: 200
- Protein: 6g
- Fat: 10g
- Carbohydrates: 24g
- Fiber: 12g
- Sugars: 10g

Serving Size: 1

Cooking Time: 5 minutes (plus overnight refrigeration)

Ingredients:

- 2 large eggs
- 1/2 cup fresh spinach, chopped
- 1/4 cup mushrooms, sliced
- 1 tablespoon olive oil
- Salt and pepper to taste

Instructions:

1. In a small bowl, whisk the eggs until well combined. Season with salt and pepper.
2. Heat the olive oil in a non-stick skillet over medium heat.
3. Add the mushrooms to the skillet and sauté for 2-3 minutes until they start to soften.
4. Add the chopped spinach to the skillet and cook for another 1-2 minutes until wilted.
5. Pour the whisked eggs over the spinach and mushrooms. Let it cook undisturbed for 2-3 minutes or until the edges start to set.
6. Using a spatula, gently lift the edges of the omelette and tilt the skillet to allow the uncooked eggs to flow underneath.
7. Cook for another 1-2 minutes until the omelette is fully set.

8. Fold the omelette in half and slide it onto a plate. Serve immediately.

Nutritional Information:

- Calories: 210
- Protein: 14g
- Fat: 16g
- Carbohydrates: 3g
- Fiber: 1g

Serving Size:

- Serves 1

Cooking Time:

- Preparation Time: 5 minutes
- Cooking Time: 10 minutes

Turmeric Golden Milk Smoothie

Ingredient:

- 1 cup unsweetened almond milk
- 1 banana
- 1 teaspoon ground turmeric
- 1/2 teaspoon ground cinnamon
- 1/4 teaspoon ground ginger
- 1 tablespoon honey or maple syrup (optional)
- 1/2 teaspoon vanilla extract
- A pinch of black pepper (to enhance turmeric absorption)
- 1/2 cup ice cubes

Instructions:

1. Add all ingredients to a blender.
2. Blend on high until smooth and creamy.
3. Pour into a glass and serve immediately.

Nutritional Information (per serving):

- Calories: 150
- Protein: 2g
- Carbohydrates: 35g

- Dietary Fiber: 3g
- Sugars: 20g
- Fat: 2g
- Saturated Fat: 0g
- Sodium: 180mg

Serving Size:

1 smoothie (approximately 12 ounces)

Cooking Time:

5 minutes

Ingredients:

- 1 cup cooked quinoa
- 1/2 cup almond milk (or any plant-based milk)
- 1 tablespoon chia seeds
- 1/2 teaspoon vanilla extract
- 1/2 cup sliced strawberries
- 1/2 cup blueberries
- 1 small banana, sliced
- 1 tablespoon honey or maple syrup (optional)
- 1/4 cup chopped nuts (almonds, walnuts, or pecans)

Instructions:

1. In a medium bowl, combine the cooked quinoa, almond milk, chia seeds, and vanilla extract. Mix well.
2. Let the mixture sit for about 10 minutes to allow the chia seeds to swell and thicken the mixture slightly.
3. Divide the quinoa mixture into two bowls.
4. Top each bowl with sliced strawberries, blueberries, and banana.
5. Drizzle with honey or maple syrup if desired.
6. Sprinkle with chopped nuts.
7. Serve immediately.

Nutritional Information (per serving):

- Calories: 350
- Protein: 10g
- Carbohydrates: 55g
- Dietary Fiber: 8g
- Sugars: 18g
- Fat: 12g
- Saturated Fat: 1g

Serving Size:

- Serves 2

Cooking Time:

- Total time: 15 minutes

Ingredient:

- 1 cup of Greek yogurt (plain, unsweetened)
- 1 tablespoon of honey
- 1/4 cup of raw almonds, chopped
- 1/2 teaspoon of cinnamon (optional)

Instructions:

- Spoon the Greek yogurt into a bowl.
- Drizzle the honey over the yogurt.
- Sprinkle the chopped almonds on top.
- If desired, add a pinch of cinnamon for extra flavor.
- Mix gently to combine the ingredients, or enjoy as is.

Nutritional Information:

- Calories: 250
- Protein: 15g
- Carbohydrates: 25g
- Fats: 10g
- Fiber: 3g
- Sugar: 15g

Serving Size:

- 1 bowl

Cooking time:

- 5 minutes

Ingredients:

- 1 medium sweet potato
- 1 ripe avocado
- 4 slices whole grain bread
- Olive oil
- Salt and pepper to taste

Instructions:

1. Preheat the oven to 400°F (200°C).
2. Wash and scrub the sweet potato thoroughly. Slice it lengthwise into 1/4-inch thick slices.
3. Place the sweet potato slices on a baking sheet. Drizzle with olive oil and season with salt and pepper.
4. Bake for 15-20 minutes, or until the sweet potato slices are tender and lightly browned.
5. While the sweet potatoes are baking, toast the bread slices until golden brown.
6. Mash the ripe avocado in a bowl and season with salt and pepper.
7. Spread the mashed avocado evenly onto each toasted bread slice.
8. Top each slice with roasted sweet potato slices.

9. Drizzle with a little more olive oil and sprinkle with additional salt and pepper if desired.

10. Serve immediately.

Nutritional Information:

- Calories per serving: 250
- Total Fat: 10g
- Saturated Fat: 1.5g
- Cholesterol: 0mg
- Sodium: 250mg
- Total Carbohydrates: 35g
- Dietary Fiber: 8g
- Sugars: 5g
- Protein: 8g

Serving Size: 4 slices

Cooking Time: 25 minutes

Ingredients:

- 1/2 cup rolled oats
- 1/2 cup almond milk (or any milk of choice)
- 1/4 cup plain Greek yogurt
- 1/4 cup fresh blueberries
- 1 tablespoon almond butter
- 1 tablespoon chia seeds
- 1 teaspoon honey (optional)
- Pinch of cinnamon (optional)

Instructions:

1. In a jar or bowl, combine rolled oats, almond milk, Greek yogurt, chia seeds, almond butter, honey, and cinnamon (if using).

2. Stir well until all ingredients are mixed thoroughly.

3. Gently fold in fresh blueberries.

4. Cover the jar or bowl with a lid or plastic wrap and refrigerate overnight, or for at least 4 hours.

5. Before serving, give the oats a good stir. If desired, add more almond milk for a creamier consistency.

6. Enjoy cold straight from the fridge, or heat in the microwave for a warm breakfast option.

Nutritional Information:

- Calories: 350
- Protein: 12g
- Carbohydrates: 45g
- Fat: 14g
- Fiber: 8g
- Sodium: 80mg

Serving Size: 1 serving

Cooking Time: 5 minutes prep + overnight chilling

Green Smoothie with Kale and
Pineapple

Ingredients:

- 1 cup chopped kale leaves
- 1 cup fresh pineapple chunks
- 1 ripe banana
- 1 tablespoon chia seeds
- 1 cup coconut water or almond milk
- Ice cubes (optional)

Instructions:

1. Add kale, pineapple chunks, banana, chia seeds, and coconut water (or almond milk) to a blender.
2. Blend until smooth and creamy. Add ice cubes if desired for a colder texture.
3. Pour into glasses and serve immediately.

Nutritional Information:

- Calories: 180
- Protein: 4g
- Carbohydrates: 35g
- Fat: 4g

- Fiber: 7g
- Vitamin C: 120% DV
- Iron: 2mg

Serving Size: 1 smoothie

Cooking Time: 5 minutes

Ingredients:

- 1 block firm tofu, drained and crumbled
- 1 red bell pepper, diced
- 1 cup spinach leaves
- 1 small onion, finely chopped
- 2 cloves garlic, minced
- 1 tbsp olive oil
- Salt and pepper to taste
- Optional: turmeric, nutritional yeast

Instructions:

1. Heat olive oil in a skillet over medium heat.
2. Add onions and garlic, sauté until softened.
3. Add bell pepper and cook until slightly tender.
4. Add crumbled tofu and stir well to combine.
5. Season with salt, pepper, and optional turmeric or nutritional yeast for flavor.
6. Cook for 5-7 minutes, stirring occasionally, until tofu is heated through and vegetables are tender.
7. Stir in spinach leaves and cook until wilted.
8. Serve hot.

Nutritional Information:

- Calories per serving: 220
- Protein: 15g
- Carbohydrates: 10g
- Fat: 14g
- Fiber: 3g

Serving Size: 2 servings

Cooking Time: 15 minutes

Ingredients:

- 1 cup buckwheat flour
- 1 tablespoon baking powder
- 1/2 teaspoon salt
- 1 tablespoon honey or maple syrup
- 1 cup almond milk (or any preferred milk)
- 1 egg
- 1 teaspoon vanilla extract
- Fresh berries (such as strawberries, blueberries, raspberries) for topping
- Maple syrup or honey (optional, for serving)

Instructions:

1. In a large bowl, whisk together buckwheat flour, baking powder, and salt.

2. In a separate bowl, whisk together honey or maple syrup, almond milk, egg, and vanilla extract.

3. Pour wet ingredients into dry ingredients and stir until just combined. Let batter sit for 5-10 minutes to thicken.

4. Heat a non-stick skillet or griddle over medium heat. Lightly grease with oil or butter.

5. Pour 1/4 cup of batter onto the skillet for each pancake. Cook until bubbles form on the surface, then flip and cook until golden brown on both sides.

6. Serve warm topped with fresh berries and a drizzle of maple syrup or honey, if desired.

Nutritional Information:

- Calories: 220 kcal
- Protein: 6g
- Carbohydrates: 40g
- Fat: 5g
- Fiber: 4g
- Sodium: 350mg

Serving Size: Makes about 8 pancakes

Cooking Time: Approximately 15 minutes

Chapter 2: Lunch Recipes

Quinoa and Roasted Vegetable Salad

Ingredients:

- 1 cup quinoa, rinsed
- 2 cups water
- 1 cup cherry tomatoes, halved
- 1 medium zucchini, diced
- 1 red bell pepper, diced
- 1 yellow bell pepper, diced
- 2 tablespoons olive oil
- 1 teaspoon dried oregano
- Salt and pepper to taste
- 1/4 cup fresh parsley, chopped
- Juice of 1 lemon

Instructions:

1. Preheat the oven to 400°F (200°C).
2. In a medium pot, bring the water to a boil. Add the quinoa, reduce the heat to low, cover, and simmer for 15 minutes or

until the water is absorbed and the quinoa is tender. Remove from heat and fluff with a fork.

3. While the quinoa is cooking, place the cherry tomatoes, zucchini, red bell pepper, and yellow bell pepper on a baking sheet. Drizzle with olive oil, sprinkle with dried oregano, salt, and pepper, and toss to coat.

4. Roast the vegetables in the preheated oven for 20-25 minutes, or until they are tender and slightly caramelized.

5. In a large bowl, combine the cooked quinoa and roasted vegetables. Add the fresh parsley and lemon juice, and toss to mix well.

6. Serve warm or chilled, as desired.

Nutritional Information:

- Calories: 240 per serving
- Protein: 7g
- Carbohydrates: 32g
- Fiber: 5g
- Fat: 10g
- Omega-3 fatty acids: 0.1g

Serving Size: 4

Cooking Time: 45 minutes

Ingredients:

- 1 salmon fillet (about 4 ounces)
- 1 tablespoon olive oil
- Juice of 1 lemon
- Salt and pepper to taste
- 1 cup broccoli florets
- 1 cup baby spinach
- 1 clove garlic, minced
- 1 teaspoon sesame seeds (optional)

Instructions:

1. Preheat the grill to medium-high heat.
2. Brush the salmon fillet with olive oil and season with lemon juice, salt, and pepper.
3. Grill the salmon for about 4-5 minutes on each side, until fully cooked and flaky.
4. While the salmon is grilling, steam the broccoli florets until tender, about 5-7 minutes.
5. In a separate pan, sauté the baby spinach and garlic with a little olive oil until wilted, about 2-3 minutes.
6. Serve the grilled salmon on a plate with steamed broccoli and sautéed spinach.
7. Sprinkle sesame seeds over the top, if using.

Nutritional Information:

- Calories: 320
- Protein: 28g
- Fat: 20g
- Carbohydrates: 6g
- Fiber: 3g

Serving Size:

- 1 serving

Cooking Time:

- 20 minutes

Ingredients:

- 1 cup dried lentils
- 1 tablespoon olive oil
- 1 onion, chopped
- 2 cloves garlic, minced
- 1 tablespoon fresh ginger, grated
- 1 teaspoon ground turmeric
- 4 cups vegetable broth
- 1 can diced tomatoes
- 1 carrot, chopped
- 1 celery stalk, chopped
- Salt and pepper to taste
- Fresh cilantro for garnish

Instructions:

1. Rinse the lentils under cold water and set aside.
2. In a large pot, heat the olive oil over medium heat. Add the onion and garlic, sauté until translucent.
3. Add the ginger and turmeric, cooking for another minute until fragrant.
4. Pour in the vegetable broth and add the lentils, tomatoes, carrot, and celery.

5. Bring to a boil, then reduce heat and simmer for 25-30 minutes, or until the lentils are tender.
6. Season with salt and pepper to taste.
7. Serve hot, garnished with fresh cilantro.

Nutritional Information:

- Calories: 230 per serving
- Protein: 12g
- Carbohydrates: 36g
- Fat: 5g
- Fiber: 12g

Serving Size:

- Serves 4

Cooking Time:

- Preparation: 10 minutes
- Cooking: 30 minutes

Ingredient:

- 1 cup canned chickpeas, drained and rinsed
- 1 ripe avocado, diced
- 1 small cucumber, diced
- 1 small red onion, finely chopped
- 1 cup cherry tomatoes, halved
- 1/4 cup fresh parsley, chopped
- 2 tablespoons olive oil
- Juice of 1 lemon
- Salt and pepper to taste

Instructions:

1. In a large bowl, combine the chickpeas, avocado, cucumber, red onion, cherry tomatoes, and parsley.
2. In a small bowl, whisk together the olive oil, lemon juice, salt, and pepper.
3. Pour the dressing over the chickpea mixture and toss gently to combine.
4. Serve immediately or refrigerate for up to 2 hours to allow flavors to meld.

Nutritional Information (per serving):

- Calories: 320
- Protein: 7g
- Carbohydrates: 26g
- Dietary Fiber: 10g
- Total Fat: 22g
- Saturated Fat: 3g
- Cholesterol: 0mg
- Sodium: 220mg

Serving Size:

2 servings

Cooking Time:

15 minutes

Ingredient:

- 1 cup cooked brown rice
- 1/2 cup diced bell peppers (any color)
- 1/2 cup chopped spinach
- 1/4 cup diced onions
- 1/2 cup diced zucchini
- 1 clove garlic, minced
- 1 tbsp olive oil
- 1 tbsp low-sodium soy sauce
- 1/2 tsp turmeric powder
- Salt and pepper to taste
- Fresh parsley for garnish (optional)

Instructions:

1. Heat the olive oil in a large skillet over medium heat.
2. Add the minced garlic and diced onions to the skillet, and sauté until the onions become translucent, about 2-3 minutes.
3. Add the bell peppers, zucchini, and turmeric powder. Stir-fry for another 5-7 minutes until the vegetables are tender.
4. Add the chopped spinach and cooked brown rice to the skillet. Stir well to combine all the ingredients.

5. Pour in the low-sodium soy sauce, and continue to stir-fry for another 2-3 minutes, ensuring the rice and vegetables are evenly coated.

6. Season with salt and pepper to taste.

7. Remove from heat and garnish with fresh parsley if desired.

8. Serve hot and enjoy a nutritious start to your day.

Nutritional Information:

- Calories: 250 per serving
- Protein: 6g
- Carbohydrates: 42g
- Fiber: 4g
- Fat: 8g
- Sodium: 300mg

Serving Size:

- Serves 2

Cooking Time:

- Total: 15 minutes

Ingredient:

- 4 bell peppers (any color)
- 1 cup fresh spinach, chopped
- 1/2 cup crumbled feta cheese
- 1/4 cup chopped onion
- 1 clove garlic, minced
- 2 large eggs
- 1/4 teaspoon black pepper
- 1 tablespoon olive oil

Instructions:

1. Preheat the oven to 375°F (190°C).
2. Cut the tops off the bell peppers and remove the seeds and membranes.
3. Heat olive oil in a skillet over medium heat. Add the onion and garlic, cooking until softened, about 3 minutes.
4. Add the chopped spinach to the skillet and cook until wilted, about 2 minutes.
5. In a bowl, whisk the eggs, then stir in the cooked spinach mixture and crumbled feta cheese. Season with black pepper.
6. Place the bell peppers in a baking dish and fill each with the egg mixture.

7. Bake in the preheated oven for 25-30 minutes, or until the eggs are set and the peppers are tender.

Nutritional Information:
- Calories: 180
- Protein: 8g
- Carbohydrates: 10g
- Fat: 12g
- Fiber: 3g

Serving Size: 4 stuffed peppers

Cooking Time: 35-40 minutes

Ingredients:

- 1 whole grain wrap
- 3 ounces of sliced turkey breast
- 1 cup fresh spinach leaves
- 1/4 cup diced tomatoes
- 1/4 cup shredded low-fat cheese
- 1 tablespoon hummus
- Salt and pepper to taste

Instructions:

1. Lay the whole grain wrap flat on a clean surface.
2. Spread the hummus evenly over the wrap.
3. Place the turkey slices on top of the hummus layer.
4. Add the fresh spinach leaves evenly over the turkey.
5. Sprinkle the diced tomatoes and shredded cheese over the spinach.
6. Season with salt and pepper to taste.
7. Carefully roll the wrap tightly, tucking in the sides as you go.
8. Slice the wrap in half and serve immediately.

Nutritional Information:

- Calories: 320
- Protein: 25g
- Carbohydrates: 30g
- Fat: 12g
- Fiber: 6g

Serving Size:

- 1 wrap

Cooking Time:

- 10 minutes

Ingredients:

- 1 medium sweet potato, peeled and diced
- 1 can (15 oz) black beans, drained and rinsed
- 1 tablespoon olive oil
- 1 teaspoon ground cumin
- 1/2 teaspoon chili powder
- 1/2 teaspoon paprika
- Salt and pepper to taste
- 4 small corn tortillas
- 1 avocado, sliced
- 1/4 cup chopped fresh cilantro
- 2 tablespoons lime juice
- 1/4 cup crumbled feta cheese (optional)

Instructions:

1. Preheat your oven to 400°F (200°C).
2. Toss the diced sweet potato with olive oil, cumin, chili powder, paprika, salt, and pepper.
3. Spread the sweet potatoes on a baking sheet and roast for 20-25 minutes, or until tender and slightly crispy.
4. In a medium saucepan, heat the black beans over medium heat until warm.

5. Warm the corn tortillas in a dry skillet or microwave until pliable.

6. Assemble the tacos by dividing the roasted sweet potatoes and black beans evenly among the tortillas.

7. Top with avocado slices, chopped cilantro, lime juice, and feta cheese if using.

8. Serve immediately and enjoy.

Nutritional Information:

- Calories: 320 per serving
- Protein: 10 grams
- Carbohydrates: 45 grams
- Fat: 12 grams
- Fiber: 12 grams
- Sugar: 6 grams

Serving Size:

- 4 tacos (1 serving is 2 tacos)

Cooking Time:

- Total: 30-35 minutes

Ingredients:

- 1 cup cooked chicken breast, shredded
- 1 cup cherry tomatoes, halved
- 1/2 cup cucumber, diced
- 1/4 cup red onion, thinly sliced
- 1/4 cup Kalamata olives, pitted and sliced
- 1/4 cup feta cheese, crumbled
- 2 tablespoons extra virgin olive oil
- 1 tablespoon lemon juice
- 1 teaspoon dried oregano
- Salt and pepper to taste
- 2 cups mixed greens (spinach, arugula, or lettuce)

Instructions:

1. In a large bowl, combine the shredded chicken, cherry tomatoes, cucumber, red onion, and Kalamata olives.
2. In a small bowl, whisk together the olive oil, lemon juice, oregano, salt, and pepper.
3. Pour the dressing over the chicken and vegetable mixture, tossing to coat evenly.
4. Add the crumbled feta cheese and gently mix to incorporate.
5. Serve the chicken salad over a bed of mixed greens.

Nutritional Information (per serving):

- Calories: 320
- Protein: 25g
- Carbohydrates: 8g
- Dietary Fiber: 3g
- Sugars: 4g
- Total Fat: 22g
- Saturated Fat: 5g
- Sodium: 480mg

Serving Size:

- 2 servings

Cooking Time:

- Preparation: 15 minutes
- Total: 15 minutes

Ingredients:

- 1 cup quinoa, rinsed
- 6 cups vegetable broth
- 1 onion, chopped
- 2 garlic cloves, minced
- 2 carrots, diced
- 2 celery stalks, diced
- 1 sweet potato, peeled and diced
- 1 cup kale, chopped
- 1 teaspoon turmeric
- Salt and pepper to taste
- Fresh parsley, chopped (for garnish)

Instructions:

1. In a large pot, heat a bit of vegetable broth over medium heat.
2. Add onion and garlic, sauté until fragrant.
3. Add carrots, celery, and sweet potato. Cook for 5 minutes.
4. Add quinoa, turmeric, and remaining vegetable broth. Bring to a boil.
5. Reduce heat and simmer for 15-20 minutes, or until quinoa and vegetables are tender.

6. Stir in kale and cook for an additional 5 minutes.

7. Season with salt and pepper to taste.

8. Serve hot, garnished with fresh parsley.

Nutritional Information:

- Calories: 250 kcal
- Protein: 9g
- Carbohydrates: 45g
- Fiber: 6g
- Fat: 4g
- Sodium: 800mg

Serving Size: 1 bowl

Cooking Time: 35-40 minutes

Chapter 3: Dinner Recipes

Baked Chicken with Sweet Potato Mash

Ingredients:

- 4 boneless, skinless chicken breasts
- 2 tbsp olive oil
- 1 tsp garlic powder
- 1 tsp paprika
- Salt and pepper to taste
- 4 medium sweet potatoes, peeled and cubed
- 1/4 cup unsweetened almond milk
- 1 tbsp butter or olive oil (optional)
- Fresh parsley, chopped (for garnish)

Instructions:

1. Preheat the oven to 400°F (200°C). Lightly grease a baking dish.
2. In a small bowl, mix olive oil, garlic powder, paprika, salt, and pepper.
3. Rub the chicken breasts with the spice mixture and place them in the baking dish.

4. Bake for 20-25 minutes or until chicken is cooked through and juices run clear.

5. While the chicken is baking, boil the sweet potatoes in a large pot of water until tender, about 15-20 minutes.

6. Drain the sweet potatoes and mash them with almond milk and butter (if using) until smooth and creamy.

7. Season with salt and pepper to taste.

8. Serve the baked chicken hot with a generous scoop of sweet potato mash.

9. Garnish with chopped fresh parsley before serving.

Nutritional Information:

- Calories: 350 per serving
- Protein: 30g
- Carbohydrates: 25g
- Fat: 15g
- Fiber: 4g
- Sodium: 450mg

Serving Size: 1 chicken breast with sweet potato mash

Cooking Time: 45 minutes

Ingredients:

- 1 block firm tofu, drained and cubed
- 1 head cauliflower, grated into rice-like pieces
- 1 red bell pepper, sliced
- 1 cup broccoli florets
- 1 carrot, thinly sliced
- 2 cloves garlic, minced
- 1 tablespoon ginger, grated
- 2 tablespoons low-sodium soy sauce or tamari
- 1 tablespoon sesame oil
- 1 tablespoon rice vinegar
- 2 green onions, chopped
- Salt and pepper to taste
- Sesame seeds for garnish

Instructions:

1. Heat sesame oil in a large skillet or wok over medium-high heat.

2. Add cubed tofu and cook until golden brown on all sides, about 5-7 minutes. Remove tofu from skillet and set aside.

3. In the same skillet, add garlic and ginger. Sauté for 1-2 minutes until fragrant.

4. Add cauliflower rice, bell pepper, broccoli, and carrot to the skillet. Stir-fry for 5-7 minutes until vegetables are tender-crisp.

5. Return tofu to the skillet. Add soy sauce (or tamari) and rice vinegar. Stir well to combine and heat through.

6. Season with salt and pepper to taste.

7. Garnish with chopped green onions and sesame seeds before serving.

Nutritional Information:

- Calories: 250
- Total Fat: 12g
- Saturated Fat: 2g
- Cholesterol: 0mg
- Sodium: 450mg
- Total Carbohydrates: 20g
- Dietary Fiber: 8g
- Sugars: 8g
- Protein: 18g

Serving Size: 1/4 of recipe

Cooking Time:

- Preparation: 15 minutes
- Cooking: 15 minutes

Ingredients:

- 4 large bell peppers (any color)
- 1 cup quinoa, cooked
- 1 can (15 oz) chickpeas, drained and rinsed
- 1 cup cherry tomatoes, halved
- 1/2 cup Kalamata olives, sliced
- 1/2 cup crumbled feta cheese
- 2 tablespoons olive oil
- 2 cloves garlic, minced
- 1 teaspoon dried oregano
- Salt and pepper to taste

Instructions:

1. Preheat oven to 375°F (190°C). Line a baking dish with parchment paper.
2. Cut the tops off the bell peppers and remove seeds and membranes.
3. In a large bowl, mix together cooked quinoa, chickpeas, cherry tomatoes, olives, feta cheese, olive oil, garlic, oregano, salt, and pepper.
4. Spoon the quinoa mixture evenly into the bell peppers.
5. Place stuffed peppers in the prepared baking dish. Cover loosely with foil.

6. Bake for 25-30 minutes, until peppers are tender.

7. Remove foil and bake for an additional 5 minutes to lightly brown the tops.

8. Serve hot, garnished with fresh herbs if desired.

Nutritional Information:

- Calories: 320 per serving
- Fat: 12g
- Carbohydrates: 42g
- Protein: 12g
- Fiber: 10g
- Sodium: 480mg

Serving Size: 1 stuffed pepper

Cooking Time: 35-40 minutes

Ingredients:

- 4 cod fillets
- 2 tablespoons olive oil
- 2 tablespoons fresh lemon juice
- 1 tablespoon chopped fresh dill
- Salt and pepper to taste

Instructions:

1. Preheat oven to 375°F (190°C).
2. Place cod fillets on a baking dish lined with parchment paper.
3. Drizzle olive oil and lemon juice over the cod.
4. Sprinkle chopped dill, salt, and pepper evenly.
5. Bake for 15-20 minutes, or until fish flakes easily with a fork.

Nutritional Information:

- Calories: 250 kcal
- Protein: 30g
- Carbohydrates: 1g
- Fat: 13g
- Fiber: 0g

- Sodium: 150mg

Serving Size: 1 cod fillet

Cooking Time: 20 minutes

Ingredients:

- 2 medium zucchinis, spiralized
- 1 cup cherry tomatoes, halved
- 1/2 cup basil pesto
- 1/4 cup pine nuts, toasted
- Salt and pepper to taste

Instructions:

1. Heat a large skillet over medium heat.
2. Add spiralized zucchini noodles and cherry tomatoes to the skillet.
3. Cook for 3-4 minutes, stirring occasionally, until zucchini noodles are tender but still crisp.
4. Stir in basil pesto until well combined.
5. Season with salt and pepper to taste.
6. Remove from heat and sprinkle with toasted pine nuts before serving.

Nutritional Information:

- Calories: 280 kcal
- Protein: 8g
- Carbohydrates: 12g

- Fiber: 4g
- Sugars: 5g
- Fat: 23g
- Saturated Fat: 4g
- Cholesterol: 8mg
- Sodium: 350mg
- Potassium: 550mg

Serving Size: 2 servings

Cooking Time: 15 minutes

Ingredients:

- 1 tbsp olive oil
- 1 onion, finely chopped
- 2 cloves garlic, minced
- 1 tsp ground cumin
- 1 tsp ground coriander
- 1/2 tsp ground turmeric
- 1/4 tsp ground cinnamon
- 1/4 tsp cayenne pepper (optional, adjust to taste)
- 1 cup diced tomatoes (canned or fresh)
- 3 cups cooked chickpeas (about 2 cans, drained and rinsed)
- 2 cups vegetable broth
- 1 cup diced carrots
- 1 cup diced sweet potatoes
- Salt and pepper, to taste
- Fresh cilantro or parsley, chopped (for garnish)

Instructions:

1. Heat olive oil in a large pot over medium heat. Add chopped onion and sauté until softened, about 5 minutes.

2. Add minced garlic, ground cumin, ground coriander, ground turmeric, ground cinnamon, and cayenne pepper (if using). Cook for another minute until fragrant.

3. Stir in diced tomatoes and cook for 2-3 minutes, allowing flavors to combine.

4. Add cooked chickpeas, vegetable broth, diced carrots, and diced sweet potatoes to the pot. Season with salt and pepper to taste.

5. Bring the stew to a boil, then reduce heat to low. Cover and simmer for 20-25 minutes, or until the carrots and sweet potatoes are tender.

6. Taste and adjust seasoning if needed. If the stew is too thick, add more vegetable broth or water to reach desired consistency.

7. Serve hot, garnished with fresh cilantro or parsley. Enjoy!

Nutritional Information:

- Calories: 280
- Total Fat: 5g
- Saturated Fat: 0.5g
- Cholesterol: 0mg
- Sodium: 580mg
- Total Carbohydrates: 50g
- Dietary Fiber: 12g
- Sugars: 10g
- Protein: 13g

Serving Size: 1.5 cups

Cooking Time: Approximately 40 minutes

Ingredients:

- 1 lb shrimp, peeled and deveined
- 1 cup quinoa, rinsed
- 2 cups water or low-sodium broth
- 1 cucumber, diced
- 1 bell pepper, diced
- 1/4 cup red onion, finely chopped
- 1/4 cup fresh parsley, chopped
- Juice of 1 lemon
- 2 tbsp olive oil
- Salt and pepper to taste

Instructions:

1. Preheat grill to medium-high heat.
2. Season shrimp with salt and pepper.
3. Grill shrimp for 2-3 minutes per side, until cooked through and slightly charred.
4. In a medium saucepan, bring water or broth to a boil. Add quinoa, reduce heat to low, cover, and simmer for 15 minutes or until quinoa is cooked and liquid is absorbed. Fluff with a fork and let cool.
5. In a large bowl, combine cooked quinoa, cucumber, bell pepper, red onion, and parsley.

6. In a small bowl, whisk together lemon juice, olive oil, salt, and pepper. Pour over quinoa salad and toss to combine.

7. Serve grilled shrimp over quinoa salad.

Nutritional Information:

- Calories: 320
- Total Fat: 10g
- Saturated Fat: 1.5g
- Cholesterol: 180mg
- Sodium: 340mg
- Total Carbohydrates: 30g
- Dietary Fiber: 4g
- Sugars: 2g
- Protein: 30g

Serving Size: 4 servings

Cooking Time: 30 minutes

Spinach and Feta Stuffed Chicken
Breast

Ingredients:

- 4 boneless, skinless chicken breasts
- 2 cups fresh spinach, chopped
- 1/2 cup crumbled feta cheese
- 1/4 cup sun-dried tomatoes, chopped
- 2 cloves garlic, minced
- Salt and pepper to taste
- Olive oil for cooking

Instructions:

1. Preheat oven to 375°F (190°C).
2. In a bowl, combine chopped spinach, feta cheese, sun-dried tomatoes, garlic, salt, and pepper.
3. Cut a pocket horizontally into each chicken breast.
4. Stuff each chicken breast with the spinach and feta mixture, pressing down gently to seal.
5. Heat olive oil in an oven-safe skillet over medium-high heat.
6. Sear stuffed chicken breasts for 3-4 minutes per side until golden brown.

7. Transfer skillet to preheated oven and bake for 20-25 minutes or until chicken is cooked through.

8. Remove from oven and let rest for 5 minutes before serving.

Nutritional Information:

- Calories per serving: 320
- Total Fat: 15g
- Saturated Fat: 6g
- Cholesterol: 120mg
- Sodium: 480mg
- Carbohydrates: 4g
- Fiber: 1g
- Sugars: 2g
- Protein: 40g

Serving Size: 1 stuffed chicken breast

Cooking Time: Approximately 35-40 minutes (including prep and baking time)

Ingredients:

- 1 cup Arborio rice
- 2 cups cubed butternut squash
- 1 small onion, finely chopped
- 2 cloves garlic, minced
- 4 cups low-sodium vegetable broth
- 1/2 cup dry white wine (optional)
- 1/4 cup grated Parmesan cheese (optional)
- 2 tablespoons olive oil
- Salt and pepper to taste
- Fresh parsley for garnish

Instructions:

1. In a large saucepan, heat olive oil over medium heat. Add onion and garlic, sauté until softened.

2. Add Arborio rice and stir to coat with oil, cooking for about 2 minutes until lightly toasted.

3. Stir in cubed butternut squash.

4. Gradually add vegetable broth, 1/2 cup at a time, stirring frequently and allowing each addition to be absorbed before adding more.

5. Continue cooking and stirring until rice is creamy and tender, about 20-25 minutes.

6. If using, stir in white wine and cook until absorbed.

7. Remove from heat and stir in Parmesan cheese if desired. Season with salt and pepper to taste.

8. Serve hot, garnished with fresh parsley.

Nutritional Information:

- Calories: 320 per serving
- Total Fat: 8g
- Saturated Fat: 2g
- Cholesterol: 5mg
- Sodium: 680mg
- Total Carbohydrate: 55g
- Dietary Fiber: 4g
- Sugars: 3g
- Protein: 6g

Serving Size: 4 servings

Cooking Time: Approximately 35 minutes

Ingredients:

- 1 tablespoon olive oil
- 1 onion, chopped
- 2 cloves garlic, minced
- 1 red bell pepper, diced
- 1 yellow bell pepper, diced
- 1 zucchini, diced
- 1 carrot, diced
- 1 cup corn kernels (fresh or frozen)
- 2 teaspoons chili powder
- 1 teaspoon cumin
- 1/2 teaspoon paprika
- Salt and pepper to taste
- 1 can (15 ounces) black beans, drained and rinsed
- 1 can (15 ounces) kidney beans, drained and rinsed
- 1 can (15 ounces) diced tomatoes
- 2 cups vegetable broth
- Fresh cilantro, chopped (for garnish)

Instructions:

1. Heat olive oil in a large pot over medium heat. Add chopped onion and minced garlic, sauté until onion becomes translucent.

2. Add diced bell peppers, zucchini, carrot, and corn kernels to the pot. Cook for about 5 minutes, stirring occasionally, until vegetables start to soften.

3. Stir in chili powder, cumin, paprika, salt, and pepper. Cook for another minute to toast the spices.

4. Add black beans, kidney beans, diced tomatoes (with juices), and vegetable broth to the pot. Bring to a boil.

5. Reduce heat to low, cover the pot, and let the chili simmer for 20-25 minutes, stirring occasionally, until vegetables are tender and flavors have melded.

6. Taste and adjust seasoning if needed. Serve hot, garnished with chopped cilantro.

Nutritional Information:

- Calories: 250 kcal
- Carbohydrates: 45g
- Protein: 12g
- Fat: 4g
- Fiber: 12g
- Sodium: 650mg

Serving Size: 1 cup

Cooking Time: 40 minutes

Chapter 6: Desserts

Dark Chocolate Avocado Mousse

Ingredients:

- Ripe avocados: 2
- Unsweetened cocoa powder: 1/2 cup
- Maple syrup or honey: 1/4 cup (adjust to taste)
- Vanilla extract: 1 teaspoon
- Almond milk or coconut milk: 1/4 cup (adjust for desired consistency)
- Dark chocolate chips (optional for garnish)

Instructions:

1. Scoop the flesh of the avocados into a blender or food processor.
2. Add cocoa powder, maple syrup or honey, vanilla extract, and almond milk.
3. Blend until smooth and creamy, scraping down the sides as needed.
4. Transfer the mousse into serving dishes.

5. Refrigerate for at least 30 minutes to allow flavors to meld.

6. Optionally, garnish with dark chocolate chips before serving.

Nutritional Information:

- Calories per serving: 220
- Total Fat: 15g
  - Saturated Fat: 4g
  - Trans Fat: 0g
- Cholesterol: 0mg
- Sodium: 10mg
- Total Carbohydrates: 25g
  - Dietary Fiber: 9g
  - Sugars: 13g
- Protein: 4g

Serving Size: 1/2 cup

Cooking Time: 10 minutes

Ingredients:

- 1 cup Greek yogurt
- 1 tablespoon honey
- 1/2 teaspoon vanilla extract
- 1/4 cup chia seeds
- 1 cup mixed berries (strawberries, blueberries, raspberries)

Instructions:

1. In a bowl, mix Greek yogurt, honey, and vanilla extract until well combined.
2. Stir in chia seeds and let the mixture sit for 10 minutes to allow chia seeds to absorb some liquid.
3. In serving glasses or bowls, layer the yogurt mixture and mixed berries.
4. Repeat layers until all ingredients are used, finishing with a layer of berries on top.
5. Refrigerate for at least 1 hour before serving to allow flavors to meld.

Nutritional Information:

- Calories: 250

- Protein: 15g
- Carbohydrates: 30g
- Fat: 9g
- Fiber: 10g

Serving Size: Makes 2 servings

Cooking Time: 10 minutes prep + 1 hour chilling time

Ingredients:

- 4 medium-sized apples (Granny Smith or Honeycrisp work well)
- 1 teaspoon ground cinnamon
- 1 tablespoon honey or maple syrup (optional)
- 1/4 cup chopped nuts (walnuts or almonds), optional
- Fresh lemon juice (from 1 lemon)

Instructions:

1. Preheat your oven to 375°F (190°C).
2. Core the apples, leaving the bottoms intact. Place them in a baking dish.
3. In a small bowl, mix together cinnamon and honey/maple syrup (if using).
4. Stuff each apple with the cinnamon mixture. If desired, sprinkle chopped nuts on top.
5. Squeeze fresh lemon juice over the apples.
6. Bake for 25-30 minutes, or until the apples are tender and lightly golden.
7. Remove from the oven and let cool slightly before serving.

Nutritional Information:

- Calories: 120 per serving
- Total Fat: 2g
- Saturated Fat: 0g
- Cholesterol: 0mg
- Sodium: 0mg
- Total Carbohydrates: 28g
- Dietary Fiber: 5g
- Sugars: 20g
- Protein: 1g

Serving Size: 1 apple

Cooking Time: 25-30 minutes

Ingredients:

- 1 cup almonds, raw and unsalted
- 1 cup shredded coconut, unsweetened
- 1/4 cup honey or maple syrup
- 1 tablespoon coconut oil
- 1/2 teaspoon vanilla extract
- Pinch of sea salt

Instructions:

1. In a food processor, pulse the almonds until finely chopped.
2. Add the shredded coconut, honey or maple syrup, coconut oil, vanilla extract, and sea salt.
3. Pulse until the mixture sticks together when pressed between your fingers.
4. Roll the mixture into small balls, about 1 inch in diameter, and place them on a baking sheet lined with parchment paper.
5. Refrigerate for at least 30 minutes to set.

Nutritional Information (per serving):

- Calories: 120
- Total Fat: 9g
  - Saturated Fat: 4g
  - Trans Fat: 0g
- Cholesterol: 0mg
- Sodium: 20mg
- Total Carbohydrates: 9g
  - Dietary Fiber: 2g
  - Sugars: 6g
- Protein: 2g

Serving Size: Makes about 12 energy balls.

Cooking Time: 10 minutes prep time + 30 minutes chilling time

Ingredients:

- 2 ripe mangoes, peeled and diced
- 1/4 cup honey or agave syrup
- Juice of 1 lime
- 1/2 cup water

Instructions:

1. In a blender, combine diced mangoes, honey or agave syrup, lime juice, and water.
2. Blend until smooth and creamy.
3. Pour the mixture into a shallow dish and freeze for 4-6 hours, stirring every hour to break up ice crystals.
4. Once frozen, scoop into serving bowls and garnish with fresh mint leaves or a slice of lime.

Nutritional Information:

- Calories: 120 per serving
- Total Fat: 0.5g
- Cholesterol: 0mg
- Sodium: 1mg
- Total Carbohydrates: 31g
- Dietary Fiber: 2g

- Sugars: 28g
- Protein: 1g

Serving Size: 1/2 cup

Cooking Time: 4-6 hours

Conclusion

In concluding your journey with the "Rheumatoid Arthritis Diet Cookbook for Women," reflect on the transformative power of nutrition in managing your health. Throughout this cookbook, you've embarked on a path toward better well-being by harnessing the healing potential of food. You've learned that diet plays a crucial role in managing rheumatoid arthritis symptoms, offering not just relief from pain but also improvements in energy levels and overall quality of life.

As you close this chapter, consider the key insights and practices you've adopted. From understanding the importance of anti-inflammatory foods to discovering delicious recipes that support joint health, each recipe and piece of advice has contributed to your holistic approach to managing rheumatoid arthritis. By embracing these dietary changes, you've empowered yourself to take control of your health and nurture your body from within.

Beyond the kitchen, this cookbook has equipped you with practical tools for navigating everyday challenges. Whether dining out, traveling, or planning meals for the week, you've learned strategies to maintain your dietary regimen while enjoying life to the fullest. These strategies have not only enhanced your physical health but also supported your emotional well-being, fostering a sense of empowerment and resilience in the face of rheumatoid arthritis.

Looking ahead, continue to integrate the lessons learned from this cookbook into your lifestyle. Embrace the variety of flavors and nutrients that each recipe offers, ensuring your meals are both nourishing and enjoyable. Stay mindful of how different foods affect your body, making adjustments as needed to support your ongoing health journey.

Remember, managing rheumatoid arthritis is a continuous process, and your dedication to a healthy diet is a cornerstone of that process. By prioritizing nutrition and making informed choices about what you eat, you are investing in your long-term health and vitality. Celebrate your progress and achievements, knowing that each meal prepared from this cookbook is a step toward a healthier, more vibrant you.

In closing, the "Rheumatoid Arthritis Diet Cookbook for Women" is more than a collection of recipes; it's a guide to living well with rheumatoid arthritis. It's a testament to your strength and determination in taking charge of your health. May this cookbook continue to inspire and support you on your journey to a life filled with health, happiness, and delicious, nourishing meals.

www.ingramcontent.com/pod-product-compliance
Lightning Source LLC
Chambersburg PA
CBHW050826250726

48653CB00006B/2444